MW00488897

happy

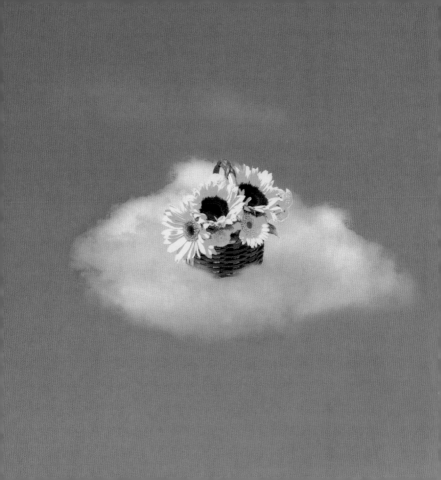

happy

100 tips to feel great

Jane Garton

BARRON'S

First edition for North America published in 2003 by Barron's Educational Series, Inc.

Copyright © **MQ Publications Ltd** 2003

All inquiries should be addressed to:
Barron's Educational Series, Inc.
250 Wireless Boulevard
Hauppauge, NY 11788
http://www.barronseduc.com

International Standard Book
No. 0-7641-5696-9

Library of Congress Catalog Card No.
2003101022

SERIES EDITOR: **Yvonne Deutch**
DESIGN: **Balley Design Associates**

Printed in China
9 8 7 6 5 4 3 2 1

For my father, with love

contents

introduction

Happiness can seem elusive, but it can be yours for good once you've found it. Your ability to enjoy life to the full is not wholly determined by your genes or your environment, despite what some people think. In fact, you can boost your happiness levels just by changing the way you view the world. Think negatively, and it's likely that things will turn out badly. But think and behave positively, and nine times out of ten the outcome will be happy.

If you want to find the joy in life, but don't know where to start, then begin right here. Dive in to the colorful pages of *HAPPY* and discover the 100 best tips on how to feel great. Take the simple act of smiling, for instance. It's now known that just lifting the corners of your mouth into a smile floods your brain with serotonin, a brain chemical that instantly enhances your mood. Simple, but effective. That's just one of the many tips that can transform your life for the better.

Best of all, happiness is incredibly infectious. That's why you should aim to spread it around. So, do yourself and your friends a favor, and get on that happiness track fast. This inspiring little book shows you how. From now on, you can look on the bright side of life and watch your life improve in leaps and bounds.

CHAPTER ONE

think happy

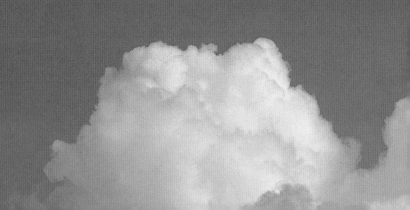

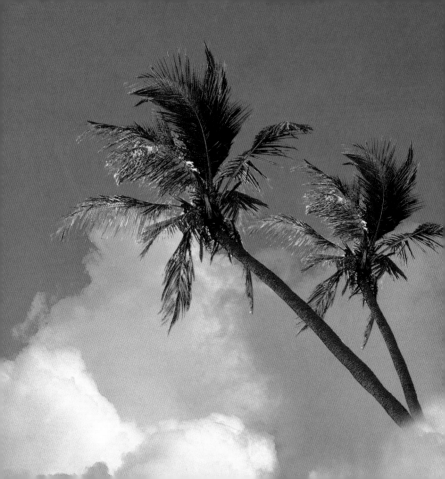

1 Lights! Action!

That sad feeling may be all in your mind. Try a session of creative visualization—it can transform your mood. Sit down quietly in a clear space and close your eyes. Now imagine yourself doing something wonderfully energetic, fun, and exciting such as leaping through the air, surfing, dancing the samba, or diving off the high board. Just "seeing" yourself in action, fizzing with energy, is often enough to bring life back to your tired mind and weary body.

2 Aim high

It's always a good idea to set yourself achievable goals, but it's even better to use the turbo power of imagination to help you get there. For example, you may decide that you'd be happier if your body was in better shape; but, instead of just thinking, "I'm going to tone and trim my waistline," bring a touch of drama to your ambition. Try rephrasing that thought into something like this: "I want to turn heads as I walk down the street and wow people when I enter a room." Remember, the more you use colorful, vibrant "wish-for-it" imagery, the easier it will be to achieve your aim and turn your dream into a reality.

3 Practice affirmations

You can't be happy if you don't like yourself, and negative thought patterns can erode your joy in life. Get yourself happy by using positive affirmation. All you need do is devise some simple phrases that encapsulate your desire to feel good. Tell yourself something like, "When I have a smile on my face, people smile back at me, I feel happy, and I always have a good day." Your affirmations should always be positive, set in the present (not the future), and describe the benefits of your action and how you feel when you do it. By repeating these positive phrases, you'll reprogram your brain into a state of mellow self-confidence.

4 Get a grip

Most situations only become stressful if
time becomes an issue. The secret is to plan
ahead and to stop leaving everything for the last
moment. Deal with letters, e-mails, phone calls, and bills
immediately. That way you remove a lot of potential
problems. Look at any possible trouble spots in your day
or week ahead and plan your time accordingly. It may mean
getting up earlier, working a little later, or saying "no" to
something, but the relief you'll feel will be well worth the extra
effort in the long run.

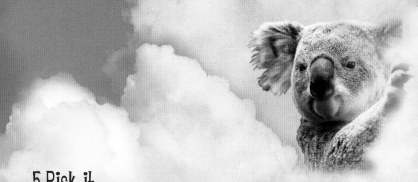

5 Risk it

If you spend most of your life in the safe and cozy zone, you'll never know what fun you're missing. Just taking one small step outside those inhibiting boundaries of security and underachievement can be liberating and uplifting. But how to take that step? One way is to take a small but deliberate risk every day. Arrange a blind date, change the color of your hair, phone someone you would like to work for and tell them so, or book yourself a solo holiday to a sunny destination. The more risks you take, the more your courage and charisma will grow. Go on, be brave—fortune favors the bold!

6 Have a nice day

You can send your happiness levels soaring by deliberately choosing to have a good day. This means adopting a "can do" attitude and putting your ball into play first, instead of always reacting to other people, or letting situations decide what happens to you. By being proactive, you make a conscious choice about what you do and don't do. Think what you can give to the day, rather than what it can give to you. Try doing this for a week and you'll be amazed how much happier and confident you feel.

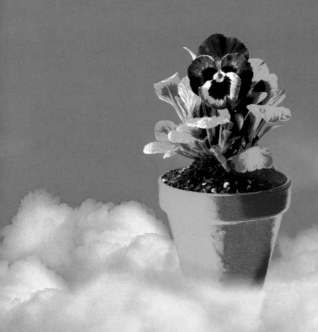

15

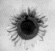

7 Learn to say the n-word

"No" is an immensely powerful word, but one that can be very difficult to say. The key is to speak with quiet assertion rather than aggression. Learn to say "no" to anything or anyone that is making you unhappy, draining your energy, or is not in your best interest. If a situation no longer enhances your life, you need to ask yourself why you are still involved. And, remember, you can still be a good friend and refuse a request. Whatever your fears and misgivings, it's likely that others will respect you even more for saying what you really feel.

8 Meditate

Deep, quiet happiness comes from a sense of inner peace. If you've never tried meditation before, you'll be amazed at the difference it can make to your mood. It's the perfect antidote to stress, and is both uplifting and calming. Learning to be still in a

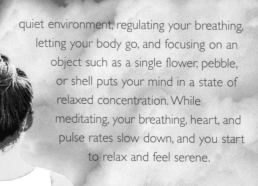

quiet environment, regulating your breathing,
letting your body go, and focusing on an
object such as a single flower, pebble,
or shell puts your mind in a state of
relaxed concentration. While
meditating, your breathing, heart, and
pulse rates slow down, and you start
to relax and feel serene.

17

9 Go with the flow

Endless repetitive activity soon takes its toll on happiness levels, and before you know it, you're so exhausted that even the simplest task becomes a giant, unhappy chore. Stop right now. Learn to just "be." Do absolutely nothing. Just sit down, or simply stop and stare. Try it for a few minutes, at least three times a day. Forget your thoughts and worries, and relish the empty moment. You'll find this helps to center you and keep you in a mood of happy balance.

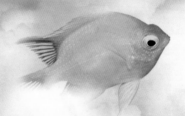

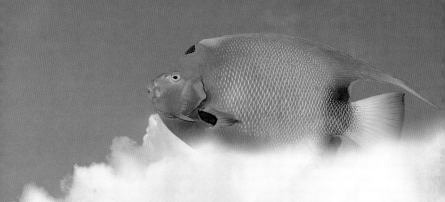

10 Decide to delegate

You might think you're indispensable, but the chances are that you're not. Trying to do everything yourself and please everyone at the same time will eventually make you feel burdened and resentful. Get out of this sad state by making a list of the tasks your partner, your children, and your colleagues can do for themselves. Then hand the tasks over quietly and firmly, and let them get on with it. Just feel that weight lift off your shoulders and enjoy a soaring sense of elation in your newfound freedom.

11 Be playful

Sometimes you feel down for no
particular reason. When you were five
years old, you'd run to your mother and say
"What can I do now?" In fact, adults need
distraction from boredom too. So, learn how
to play; do something completely absorbing—
solve a jigsaw puzzle, paint a picture, water your
plants, organize your photograph album, or
rearrange your cabinets. Anything that keeps your
mind active and preoccupied should do the trick.

12 Wise up

Standing back and analyzing how you are
really spending your days can lead to new
beginnings and a happier life. It also means

asking yourself some tough questions. Are you truly doing what you want? Is your job satisfying? Are you happy with your relationships? Are you fulfilling your potential? If what you are doing goes against your inner values, think of ways in which you can start changing things for the better. A sure way to make dreams come true is to start living them now.

13 Decisions decisions

Making a rational choice is satisfying, because the clearer you are about decisions, the better. But you shouldn't always be ruled by your head. You usually know when something "feels" wrong, even though logic suggests it's a good idea. In fact, you'll probably be happier when you follow your instincts; they stem from your deepest self, beyond the influence of family and friends. So, if you feel something or someone could make you happy, although it may seem irrational, trust yourself, go for it, and enjoy.

14 Follow that star

Next time you find yourself in a situation you dread, think of a person who has the confidence and bravura to deal with it. Now imagine how your role model would handle tough moments with your boss or bank manager, say, and take your cue from that. Rehearse a few outrageously dramatic scenes in your mind—this can be highly entertaining, as well as calming—and view your problems from a more humorous perspective.

15 Don't worry

Worrying never got anyone anywhere, and it certainly won't make you happy. So how about doing something about your worries instead of just obsessing about them? Get a piece of paper and make a list of what's bugging you, in order of priority. Nine times out of ten, seeing your troubles written down on paper helps you to view them in a new light.

16 Look ahead

Often, you wish you had done something differently; but it's pointless to regret the past: what's done is done and can't be changed. You probably did the best you could, so blaming yourself is a waste of energy. From now on, switch your thoughts to the future and start to think ahead positively. It's far better to direct your efforts into events you can influence: learn from past mistakes, and at the same time, create a bright and happy future.

17 Forgive and forget

If a friend has upset you, let your resentment go. It's normal to feel angry and want revenge, but it won't help your stress levels. It's better to move on, and be gracious, rather than harboring a grudge. If you find this hard, imagine how you'd feel if you knew this was the last time you'd ever see your friend? That one thought will show how important it is to forgive and forget.

18 Walk tall

Stop comparing yourself with other people to your own detriment. However wonderful others may seem compared to you, be assured that every great looking person knows that there's always someone more attractive than him or her. So, instead of putting yourself down, look up to yourself. Remember, real joy comes from within. You are a complete original; happiness is accepting yourself as you are.

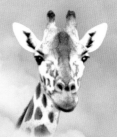

19 Get a sense of direction

Drifting aimlessly through your life is a surefire recipe for unhappiness and dissatisfaction. What you need is a realistic action plan. Take a couple of hours and compile a list divided into long-term and short-term goals for yourself. These are unique to you—they may range from cutting down on chocolate to taking up a new career. Start with the smaller goals, take each one in turn, and make a detailed action plan to drive you forward. Pin up your list where you can see it, and get to work on your first target. As you accomplish each stage, you'll experience a happy glow of personal achievement.

20 See the bigger picture

The secret of staying happy despite the
vagaries of life's ups and downs is to cultivate
a sense of perspective. Depressed people tend to
"catastrophize" upsetting events, telling themselves they are
the worst things that ever occurred. Instead of doing this, step
back from the cause of your stress and unhappiness. Ask
yourself "How will this situation look in a week, a month, a year,
five years?" In most cases, you'll soon see that it isn't important
in the grand scheme of things.

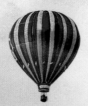

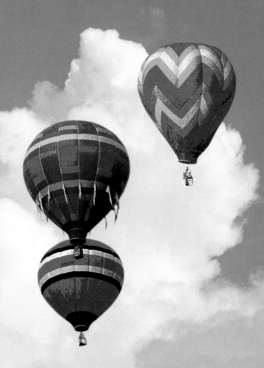

CHAPTER TWO

get happy

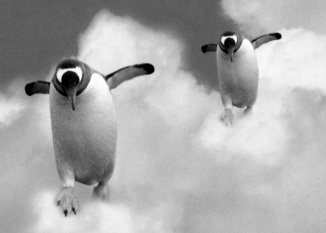

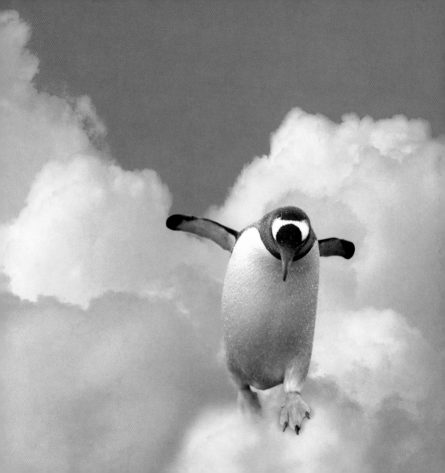

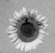

21 Get high on love

There are various reasons why making love makes you so happy—some of these are to do with the intricacy of your body's biochemistry. During tender moments, the pathways in your brain become intoxicated with raised levels of dopamine and other, natural chemicals of love. As the brain revs up for sex, the production of stress hormones such as cortisol drops dramatically. The result is a long, glorious natural high.

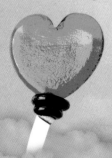

22 Shake it

A modest amount of regular daily exercise can do wonders for your mood. It produces endorphins, the body's own feel-good hormones, and also raises levels of brain chemicals such as serotonin, the "happiness hormone." Just 20 minutes of simple activity at least three times a week will do the magic trick—for instance, climb the stairs instead of taking the elevator, walk to the shops instead of using the car, and take the dog for a nice long run. Result? A happy, healthy person in no time at all.

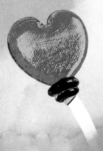

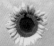

23 Happy face

This easy five-minute facial massage will raise your spirits and stimulate your senses.

- Place your fingers on the center of your forehead, press, and hold for five seconds.
- Move them to your temples, circle several times, press, and hold for five seconds.
- Lightly place two fingers on either side of your nose, press, and hold for five seconds; then move down, pressing under your cheekbones, and hold for five seconds.
- Place your fingers under your ears, circle several times, press, hold for five seconds, and repeat the circling move.

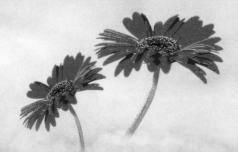

24 Take Flowers

Be prepared for tricky moments with a stock of Bach Flower remedies. They work by changing the emotions from negative to positive, and there's a potion to suit most moods:

Beech for constantly finding fault with others

Cerato for lack of confidence

Crab Apple for cleansing and self-hatred

Elm for a sense of overwhelming responsibility

Holly for negative feelings such as hatred or envy

Hornbill for extra energy

Rock Rose for terror and fright

Star of Bethlehem for shock

Wild Rose for drifting, resignation, apathy

Rescue remedy a good standby for moments of crisis such as shock, fear, panic, emotional upsets, and exam nerves.

Put two drops of your chosen remedy in a glass of water and sip four times a day.

25 Sleep well

Get eight hours' sleep a night, and you're much more likely to
start the day in a happy frame of mind. As well as keeping you
on an even keel emotionally, it will boost your immune system
and help you to think more clearly. Try the following sleep-
promoting tips:

- Go to bed and get up at the same time.
- Avoid caffeine and alcohol a few hours before bedtime.
- Make love—it will send you to sleep in a lovely, happy mood.
- Keep your bedroom well ventilated.
- If sleep evades you, don't just lie there. Get up and do
  something, but make sure it's quiet and relaxing.

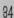

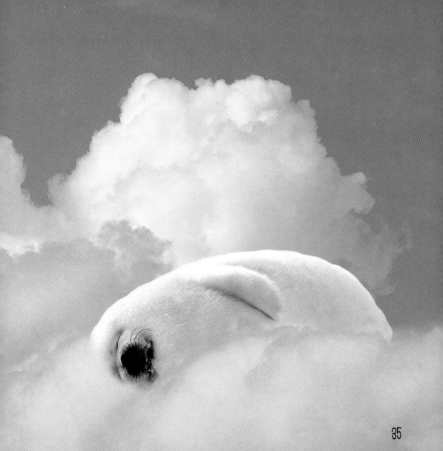

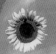

26 Brush up

If you're feeling sluggish, and your body is crying out for
stimulation, a daily session of skin brushing will perk you up. With
a hemp glove or a long-handled natural bristle brush, brush your
feet and up your legs with long, sweeping strokes. Then move on
to your buttocks and lower back, always working in the direction
of your heart. Now brush the front and back of each hand, up
your arms, across your shoulders, and down your chest. Do your
abdomen last, with clockwise, circular movements. The whole
routine should take around five minutes, or as long as it takes to
run your bath.

27 Remedy it

Known for its subtle power, homeopathy can uplift the body and
soul. Try the following remedies and feel your spirits rise: choose
Nux Vomica if you are overworked and tired out; Calc Carb if

even the slightest physical or mental exertion exhausts you, or you develop an aversion to effort; Sepia for apathy and lack of interest in anything, including sex; and Carbo Veg (known as the "corpse reviver") if you are close to collapse or have no interest in life. Remedies should be taken in the 6c potency, according to instructions on the bottle.

28 Scalped

If you tend to store tension in your head, here's a scalp massage to ease the strain. Find your hairline, and, using four fingertips of both hands, press your forehead for a couple of seconds, then release. Following your hairline from front to back, continue this movement around your head. Repeat the circuit two or three times. Finish off by pressing your fingertips into the crown of your head. It takes just a few seconds, and best of all, the happy benefits are instant.

29 Sing out

Think how wonderfully elated you feel after standing in a crowd, singing along at the top of your voice. Well, the good news is, you can sing to your heart's content at any time you choose and still reap the feel-good benefits. All you have to do is put on your favorite tune, at home or in the car, and sing out. Singing boosts happiness because it makes you breathe deeper, which means more oxygen reaches your muscles, and you start to relax and wind down.

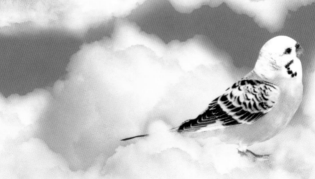

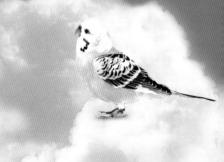

30 Take a deep breath

Often there's no escaping those tense, anxious moments, but knowing how to breathe properly can help alleviate the strain. Stand or sit with your weight evenly distributed. Put one hand on your abdomen and the other on your chest. Breathe deeply and slowly through your nose. Try to make your "out" breath longer than your "in" breath, and pull in your abdomen as you exhale. If your chest is moving more than your stomach, you're not breathing correctly. Practice for a few moments each day.

31 Sunny side up

Do you know why you feel so much happier on a sunny day? As light enters the eye, it sends electrical impulses to the brain; these trigger the hypothalamus gland, which regulates most of the body's automatic functions, including mood. The more light, the better your mood. Make sure your home and your workplace receive as much light as possible. If either is on the dark side, it might be worth considering using daylight bulbs, or even a light box, to make sure you get your daily fix.

32 Stretch yourself

They say that stretching is a wake-up call for the body, and there's really nothing like it for lifting your spirits. So, before you get going on your day, set aside five minutes for a good stretch. Start by reaching above your head as high as you can with your fingertips. Then shrug your shoulders up and down from your ears, clasp your hands behind your back to release shoulder blade tension, and have a good yawn. This series of movements increases oxygen flow to the brain, which in turn stimulates the production of endorphins, the body's own feel-good hormones.

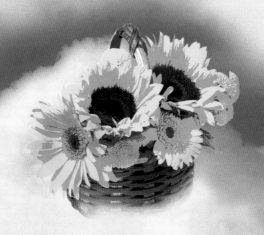

33 Reflex action

Reflexology is a natural mood boost you must not miss. The points or reflexes are manipulated by firm pressure, not light, fluttery movements; it won't tickle, but you'll feel like smiling. You can book a session with a professional, or try this simple tip to give you an instant happiness charge: find the reflex point at the base of the ball of your foot, just beneath your big toe (it relates to your adrenal glands). Using your thumb or finger, push down steadily and, keeping the pressure on the point for about 30 seconds, "walk it" by moving your wrist up and down. It may sound difficult, but with practice, it will become second nature.

34 Happy mood music

Want to change your mood from negative to positive? Then try some music therapy. The key is to observe exactly how you feel and gradually shift your mood by a careful choice of tunes. If you're feeling low, start with something slow and soothing, then follow with a more uplifting tune, and, as a grand finale, try something rousing like the "Hallelujah" chorus from Handel's *Messiah*. Invest in a personal stereo, and you can plug into this instant mood-lifter wherever you are.

35 Press here for happiness

Follow in the steps of the ancient gurus of the East and massage away your cares with some soothing acupressure. You don't have to be an expert to give yourself an amazing mood lift. Try this simple procedure to boost your happiness levels. Find the acupressure point in the fleshy part of your hand between your thumb and forefinger, and press firmly down with the ball of your thumb or the tips of your fingers. Hold for about 20 seconds, then let go slowly and gently. Wait for 10 seconds, and then repeat the move up to five times.

36 Shower the blues away

Get your day off to a happy start with an uplifting wake-up shower. Alternating blasts of cold and hot water will kick start your metabolism and boost your circulation, encouraging oxygen-rich blood to reach every tissue of your body. To continue the feel-good feeling, pat yourself dry with a thick, fluffy towel and moisturize your skin from head to toe with a body cream enriched with a few drops of peppermint or pine essential oil.

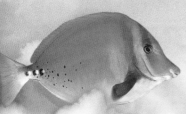

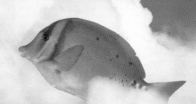

37 Dancing school

You may aspire to an organized dance class, but when you're in need of an instant cheer fix, a better (and cheaper) option is to put on your favorite music and get moving right there in your living room. Play something with a strong rhythm, and let your body leap, bend, twist, and spin to the beat. Do whatever comes naturally. There's no pressure to move in a specific way. When you're all tired out, simply lie down on the floor for a few moments to let your heartbeat slow down and enjoy the feeling of contentment that floods your soul.

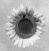

38 Essentially happy

When the going gets tough, let the sweet aroma of essential oils soothe your senses. Working on the limbic system in the brain, the area associated with moods and emotions, the scents you instinctively prefer tend to make you feel happier about life.

Experiment a little: try peppermint to revive, lemongrass to wake you up, orange to lighten your mood, and lavender to calm you down; or blend a mixture of oils. Add five drops of the essential oil to an almond carrier oil, and use in a burner, or drip your favorite essential oil onto your handkerchief.

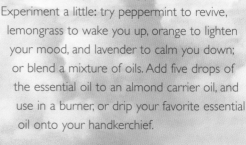
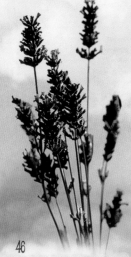
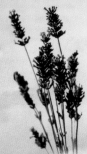

39 Blissed out bath

Happiness is a relaxing, pampering bath scented with soothing herbs, especially when you're feeling in need of some tender loving care. Camomile, lavender, lime flowers, lemon balm, or passion flower are all good choices. Steep the herbs in hot water, strain, allow to cool, and add the liquid to your bath. Alternatively, wrap them in a cheesecloth or muslin bag and hang it from the running faucet, so the water runs through as your bath fills up. Lie back and relax for 20 minutes before toweling yourself dry and drifting off to bed for a long, happy sleep.

40 Relax, relax, relax

If work or family pressures are getting the better of you, this quick relaxation exercise will help to keep you on the right side of sanity. It can be done anywhere, but start by practicing it in your own home for around 20 minutes a day. Tense and relax all the major muscle groups in your body in turn. Start with your feet, and work your way up your legs, buttocks, spine, shoulders, arms, hands, chest, and abdomen, finishing with the muscles in your head and face. Focus on the different sensation between tension and relaxation.

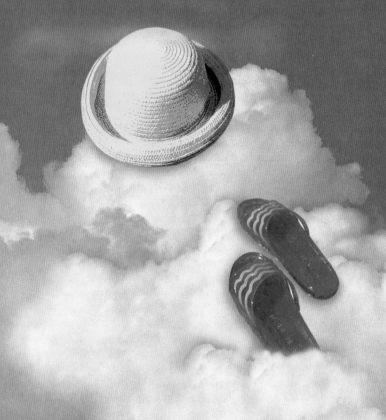

CHAPTER THREE

happy food

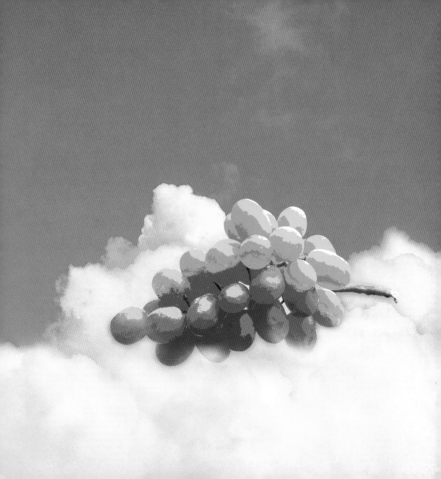

41 Watermelon detox

You won't be happy if you're feeling sluggish day after day;
but a short, sharp, 24-hour detox may be just what you
need to revive your spirits and restore all that vigor.
Constant tiredness can mean that your liver is suffering
from toxin overload and is in need of a rest. So, eating
system-cleansing fruit such as watermelon (or grapes) for a
day may give it the break it needs. You will benefit even
more if you eat plain foods such as vegetables, fish,
and rice the day before and the day after your
detox. And don't forget to drink at least
eight to ten 8oz glasses of water
to flush out the toxins.

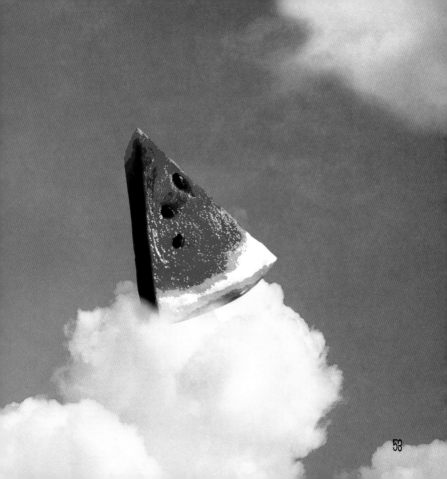

42 Spice it up

If your moods are unpredictable, spicing up your diet with hot foods could help to put them on a more even keel. Chili peppers stimulate the circulation and contain capsaicin, a substance known to boost endorphins, the body's own natural feel-good hormones. Cayenne pepper is a great restorative and digestive aid. A few drops in a cup of herbal tea will perk you up and give you a warm glow. And ginger, the most versatile of spices, is also great for stimulating the senses. Use it generously to flavor your food.

43 Breakfast like a king

It's tempting to skip breakfast when you're in a hurry, but that's a bad idea. Eating an energizing breakfast instantly reduces the likelihood of a mid-morning slump, and flagging happiness levels later in the day. Here are some suggestions:

- A glass of unsweetened fruit juice. Choose citrus-based varieties that are rich in Vitamin C.
- A bowl of whole grain, fiber-rich cereal such as muesli with semi-skimmed or skimmed milk.
- A slice of wholemeal or granary toast spread with a low-fat butter or margarine, natural peanut butter, or yeast extract.

44 Supplementary benefits

However good your diet, it can be difficult to get the right amount of nutrients needed for a healthy, balanced life from the food you eat. If you think your diet could be lacking, taking supplements is the best way to make up for any shortfall. Start off with a good all-around multivitamin or try one of the following to perk you up: co-enzyme Q10, Vitamin C, selenium, or any of the B vitamins. Adding spirulina or wheat germ powder to your morning smoothie can also give an extra energy boost.

45 Get well oiled

Although fats should take up no more than 20 percent of your overall diet, some essentially fatty acids such as omega 6 oils can help to keep energy levels high by regulating your metabolism. They also boost your immune system and make you strong enough to fight infection. Rich sources of omega 6 oils include corn, sesame, and unrefined safflower and sunflower oils, so use these regularly for cooking and in salad dressings.

46 Drink up

Feeling tired and low can be debilitating, but the happy answer to your problem could lie in a simple glass of water. Most of us don't drink nearly enough, but water is needed for the smooth functioning of every single bodily process. Aim to drink at least eight to ten 8oz glasses of water a day, and you'll soon see the difference. For starters, it banishes headaches caused by dehydration, flushes out toxins, and plumps up cells, making your skin and hair glow. If you find plain water boring, zip it up with a slice of orange or lemon, a sliver of ginger, or a sprig of mint.

47 Juice it

One of the easiest ways to get more vitality into your daily life is to drink freshly-made juices packed with the life force of plants—vitamins, minerals, enzymes, and energizing natural fruit sugars. Try different mixes such as green apple and watermelon, orange and strawberry, grape, apricot, passion fruit and mango, cucumber, beetroot and tomato, or avocado, carrot, and orange. Drink them on their own, or blend them with bananas, soy milk, or yogurt to make a delicious smoothie.

48 Herbal boosters

Stress is the biggest happiness buster of all and can really sap your energy. But, luckily, there's a special group of herbs, known as adaptogens, that can help you through those challenging times. Try a Chinese ginseng supplement, which boosts metabolism and helps normalize body systems, including glucose production.

Ginseng has been in uninterrupted use in China for over 2,000 years. Siberian ginseng is reputed to be the best choice. Known as "the king of all tonics," it is stimulating and restorative, and can help improve stamina, strength, alertness, and concentration. Students use it to achieve better results and shift nurses to adapt from day to night work.

49 Take five

We all know that eating five portions of fruit and vegetables every day will give us the necessary nutrients to help us deal with the daily grind, as well as fight disease, but many of us still find it difficult to make it a regular routine. To help you fit them in, try this: have one piece of fruit at breakfast, a generous salad at lunchtime and fresh fruit for dessert, a piece of fruit in the middle of the afternoon, and two or three vegetables at dinner, followed by another generous portion of fruit.

50 Kick the caffeine

They may give you an instant boost, but caffeine-laden drinks such as coffee, tea, and cola can make you jittery and more exhausted in the long term. Caffeine stimulates the stress hormone adrenaline, which explains the quick lift, but it also decreases the effect of a calming brain chemical that regulates the production and storage of energy. Also, caffeine doesn't stay in the body for long; hence, that sluggish feeling and craving for another fix as the effects wear off. Switching to decaffeinated coffee, or better still, herbal teas or water, will help to keep your mood on a more even keel.

51 Take tea

Once you've kicked the caffeine habit, it can be difficult to know what to sip instead. We all like variety, and that's where the dazzling range of herbal teas comes to your aid. Take a few minutes to explore the herbal tea counter at your local supermarket or health store; you'll be amazed at the range of flavors and varieties available. As well as being caffeine-free, herbal teas can quench your thirst and lift your spirits much faster than traditional tea. Try peppermint to revive and invigorate, camomile to calm you down, or ginseng to energize and stimulate. If you're feeling bloated or sluggish, try nettle or fennel tea, as both are natural diuretics.

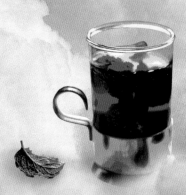

52 Indulge yourself

A little of what you enjoy can do you good, especially if it's a
small piece of chocolate. This tempting treat contains a chemical
called theobromine, which helps to increase your levels of
endorphins, the body's own feel-good hormones. It also contains
polyphenols; these help to prevent harmful cholesterol building
up in the arteries, thereby reducing the risk of heart disease.
Always choose good quality, dark chocolate, as it is more likely to
contain higher levels of pure cocoa, as well as less fat and sugar.
Remember, moderation is the key—you only need a little.

53 Cheers!

The health dangers of alcohol go without saying, but there's
evidence that a glass of red wine with your supper may be
beneficial. It can aid digestion, and relax you if you're feeling
stressed. Research also shows it contains substances that may

help to thin your blood, and so reduce your risk of heart disease. But don't go overboard. Remember, if you drink alcohol in large quantities, it will upset virtually every metabolic process, making you less able to cope with life mentally and physically. It is also high in calories and can lead to weight gain.

54 Watch that sugar

If you find your moods swing up and down like a yo-yo, too much, or too little, blood sugar could be the culprit. The best way to avoid these highs and lows is to go for foods that release sugar evenly throughout the day. Good choices include grains and vegetables that contain complex carbohydrates, combined with a small amount of protein from animal foods, dairy products, nuts, and seeds. Limit your intake of biscuits, cakes, and sweets—they may give you an instant sugar rush, making life seem brighter, but the effects will only be temporary.

55 Get grazing

Think how young children eat little and often to fuel their action-packed lives. They usually have boundless reserves of energy, and are raring to go for hours at a time. If you have blue moments during the day, you might try taking a leaf out of the same book and eat a small snack every few hours. This will help to keep your metabolism ticking over, supply your body with a constant stream of glucose so you don't get energy highs and lows, and reduce stress on your digestive system. Quick, easy, energy-boosting snacks to choose include almonds, chopped dates, an apple, sugar-free cereal bars, oat cake with cottage cheese, or fruit topped with sesame seeds.

56 Eat natural

If you want to get happy, forget processed or refined foods. Chances are they're full of sugar, fat, and additives that don't score high on the well-being chart. Instead, go for plenty of home-cooked whole foods such as grilled fish, fresh fruit, and vegetables. These are rich in antioxidant vitamins and minerals that help build up immunity, and protect against long-term lows. They're also full of natural flavor, so you'll enjoy eating them.

57 Shop happy

Stocking up with mood-boosting foods will help to put you on the fast track to happiness. Make sure you include plenty of the following on your weekly supermarket list—fish, turkey, chicken, cottage cheese, beans, avocados, bananas, and wheat germ. All these foods contain natural tryptophan, which can boost levels of serotonin, the brain chemical that helps keep your mood mellow. Other staples to drop in the shopping trolley are green vegetables, nuts, pulses, potatoes, and wholemeal bread. They're all good sources of magnesium, which is needed by your body to manufacture dopamine, another mood-enhancing chemical.

58 Pump some iron

Feeling dispirited and lacking in energy could mean that your iron levels are at an all-time low. A good intake of iron helps the blood carry oxygen around the body and makes you more alert, while a deficiency can lead to listlessness. To keep your levels up, make sure your diet includes plenty of iron-rich foods such as liver, sardines, whole grains, kidney beans, leafy green vegetables, and at least one portion of pulses a day. Alternatively, you might try taking an iron supplement—you can buy one from your local pharmacy or health store.

59 Enjoy your oats

For a quick mood boost, choose oat-based cereal bars naturally sweetened with fruit and honey. Oats are brimming with slow-release energy thanks to their soluble fiber—a gummy substance that slows down absorption and digestion, giving you a long-lasting high. They are also rich in B vitamins, needed by your body to use the energy it gets from food. Oats are also said to help boost sexual energy levels; hence, the popular saying about sowing your wild oats.

60 Lunch anyone?

A good lunch lifts your spirits, and can give you a great energy boost to take you through the afternoon. But what if your typical reaction is to feel sleepy and irritable a couple of hours later? The answer is to choose your midday menu carefully. Avoid eating large helpings of carbohydrate-rich foods such as bread, pastry, or pasta; instead, look for light, appetizing dishes such as sushi, Caesar salad, or a tuna salad. If you want something hot, choose a fragrant, warming soup made from fresh ingredients. Dessert? Easy—just have some fresh fruit, or even a slice of fruit pie (but skip the cream).

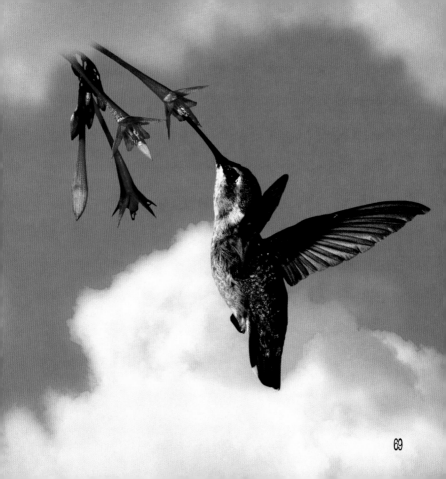

CHAPTER FOUR

simply happy

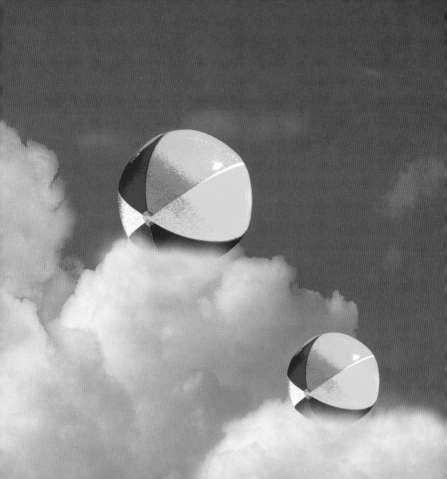

61 Pat a pet

Spending time with your pets brings you
countless happy moments, as well as being good for
your health. Patting a dog has been shown to lower your
heart rate and calm you down, while stroking a purring cat in
your lap can work wonders if you are feeling stressed. Gazing at
vistas of tranquil underwater life is also great for your mood—as
you watch fish swimming around in a tank, your brain waves
switch over to deep relaxation alpha mode. Even if you haven't
got the real thing, don't despair. It's now thought that stroking
soft, furry toys can have a similar effect—so get happy by giving
your teddy bear a pat.

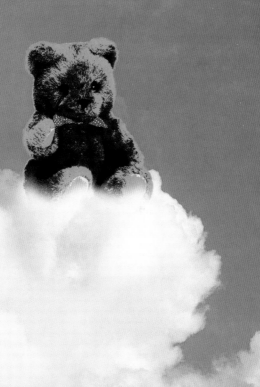

62 Have a good laugh

Three minutes of good, hearty, rip-roaring laughter can be as
beneficial to your body as ten minutes of hard aerobic exercise.
It deepens your breathing, lifts levels of endorphins, the body's
own feel-good hormones, and protects you against depression.
So, if you want to feel happy and bubbly, get those laughter
hormones going—see a funny film, read a funny book, think back
to a funny occasion, and have a really good chuckle. Giggling also
gives facial muscles a good workout and will make everyone
around you feel better, too.

63 Brighten someone's day

Think how special you feel when someone gives up their seat for
you in a crowded train or offers to carry your heavy shopping
bags. It can put you in a good mood for the rest of the day.
Interestingly, this feel-good factor works both ways—you also feel

happy and pleased when you've done something nice for another person. This is an example of positive social feedback in action; a smile, a friendly word, or just simply saying "please" and "thank you" can make all the difference to the other person's mood. And their delighted response makes your life happier too.

64 Take a mind trip

Give yourself a treat and take a perfect vacation in your mind. Create a mental picture of your dream holiday. Choose a really beautiful setting—it might be by the sea, in the mountains, or in the forest. Fill the scene with as much color and detail as you can. Imagine the scent of the flowers and foliage, the warmth of the sun on your skin, the sound of waves crashing on the rocks, or the colors of a beautiful sunset. Focus on these vivid images for up to 15 minutes. Then, slowly let the image go. When you open your eyes, you'll be amazed how happy you feel.

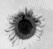

65 See red

Red is the most vivid, vibrant color in the spectrum and is also one of the best mood-boosters—it's no coincidence that the phrase "painting the town red" is connected with wild celebrations. Try it yourself: put on a red shirt, wear a red hat, try a bright red lipstick, paint your nails scarlet, buy a bunch of red roses, or throw a bright red cushion onto your favorite chair, and watch your spirits soar. Other "happy"

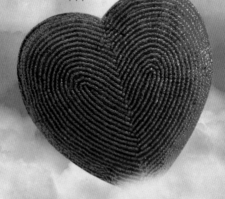

colors to include in your life are: yellow to stimulate the mind, blue to relax you and help you sleep, violet for stress and anxiety, and green, which is calming, and also has a tonic effect.

66 Have fun

Being silly, sharing a good joke, or fooling around is not just for kids. Taking life a little less seriously can be wonderfully invigorating and uplifting, whatever your age. Pretend you're a child for a moment—tell a "knock-knock" joke, start a water fight, throw pillows at your partner, splash about in the puddles, blow a few bubbles, or try catching leaves in the park. Isn't that fun? Don't worry about what others might think. If it makes you feel happy, that's all that matters. Just do it.

67 Brain workout

Your brain is just like any other muscle in your body; it needs
stretching and stimulating on a daily basis to keep it fit and happy.
So, make a new resolve to shake up your synapses by learning
four new things every day—these can be your friends' car license
plate numbers, home addresses, a new joke, an interesting quote,
or a complex phone number—anything that grabs your
attention. You may enjoy solving crossword puzzles, reading a
book, or playing board games, for instance. The idea is to keep
your brain absorbed and attentive. This will stave off mind-
deadening boredom—the archenemy of happiness.

68 Have a catnap

A few moments sleep in the afternoon may seem like the
ultimate indulgence, but it can make you happy and alert for the
rest of the day. The best times for napping are between 2 P.M.

and 4 P.M.—any later and you could risk having trouble getting to sleep at bedtime. Here's how to nap: find a comfortable chair, or put a cushion on your desk, and rest your head on it. Set an alarm for 20 minutes, close your eyes, and relax. Don't nap for longer than this, as you could fall into a deep sleep and feel groggy on waking.

69 A tonic effect

Give your system a spring cleaning! A bunch of red grapes, a fresh garlic clove (or an odorless garlic capsule), a glass of carrot or beetroot juice, or a cup of dandelion or fennel tea are simple and effective. Alternatively, try the following tonic on a daily basis for three weeks (you can get the ingredients from health stores). Mix together 1 tablespoon of aloe vera juice, 1 teaspoon of liquid chlorophyll, and 1 teaspoon of psyllium husk in a glass of cold water. Drink immediately, preferably 20 minutes before breakfast.

70 Say it with flowers

Brighten up your day and fill your house with sweet-scented flowers, or send a meaningful bunch to a friend, to bring some happy moments. Choose from the following according to your mood: bluebells for constancy, buttercups for cheerfulness, carnations for affection, chrysanthemums for friendship, daisies for innocence, forget-me-nots for true love, honeysuckle for devotion, lilies for beauty, poppies for consolation, red roses for undying love, sweet peas for gratitude, or violets for fidelity.

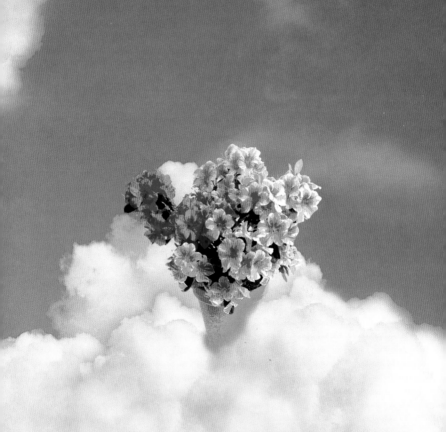

71 Watch the clouds go by

More money, a fancy car, or a new home may seem attractive, but, according to the experts, these only go so far when it comes to making you happy. However, simpler pleasures—watching bees gather pollen, walking through the park on a summer's day, listening to the crashing waves, playing with your kids, basking in

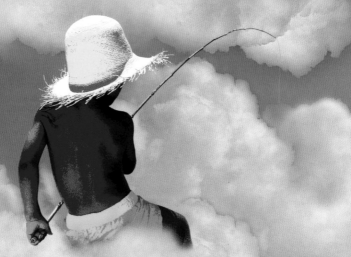

the sunshine—can bring lasting joy. Try to spend some time every day just enjoying what life has to offer for free.

72 Touch me

When was the last time you gave someone a hug? Perhaps you could you do with one yourself right now. Of all our senses, touch is one of the most neglected, and that's so sad. A simple hug or cuddle releases endorphins, the body's own feel-good hormones, as well as serotonin, another natural feel-good substance. Touch also stimulates a surge of oxytocin, sometimes dubbed the love chemical. This increases sensitivity and is active in sexual and parental bonding. The advice is simple: touch and be touched at every opportunity—it can truly enhance your health and happiness.

73 Phone a friend

If you are having a bad day, you may be tempted to stay at home and brood. But wallowing in your depression and feeling sorry for yourself is the worst thing you can do. Instead, pick up the phone and call your friends and family. They are your support network. It's far better to talk about what's worrying you, and often sharing problems with someone else makes you see them in a different light. And who knows? The day may go on to have some happy moments.

74 Take the sunny side

As soon as the sun starts to shine, snatch as many happy moments outdoors as you can. Sunlight helps to boost levels of serotonin, the feel-good chemical that helps to keep your mood equable and balanced. Sunlight is also essential for the manufacture of Vitamin D, which the body needs for healthy bones and nerves. It's not just body chemistry that makes you feel better when the sun comes out, however. The warmth also encourages you to relax and unwind and to eat lighter, healthier meals that will lead to a happier you in the long run.

75 Dress up

Think how good it feels to dress up for a special occasion; you get such pleasure from fixing your hair just right and making yourself look your best. But why reserve that delightful feeling for parties or dinner dates? It may be just another day in the office, or a routine morning taking junior to school, but if you're wearing pretty lingerie, your most attractive outfit, and heels to die for, you'll feel proud to be looking your best. Moreover, when you're feeling fine and dandy, you come over as happy and confident. This, in turn, generates waves of appreciative feedback—people respond most positively when you're pleased with yourself.

76 Calm waters

Water can have miraculous, mood-changing qualities. When you're feeling stressed and mentally exhausted, just head for the nearest stretch of water and regain your peace of mind. It can be a small pond, lake, river, or stream—the effect will be the same. Just walk quietly alongside, or sit and gaze into the water, letting your stress dissolve into the depths. As your racing thoughts retreat into the background, you'll gradually feel lulled and calmed—this is because looking deep into water changes the pattern of your brain waves. For many people, a simple session of water gazing is a powerful therapeutic experience—so it's a good strategy if you've never tried it for yourself.

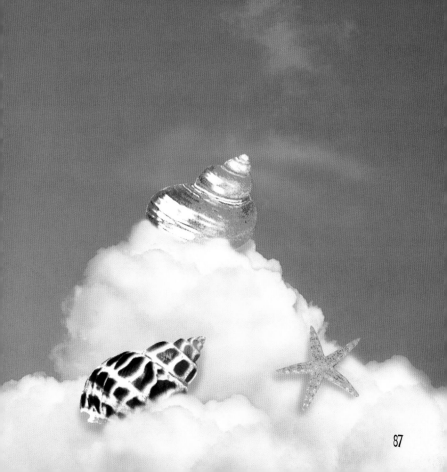

77 Happy screensavers

Taking photographs of friends and family, an inspiring landscape, or some awesome architecture can bring you hours of happy fun. And that's not all. When your shots are developed, why not scan your favorites and make an instant screensaver for your computer. This way, every time you return to the menu, or switch on or off, you will be greeted by smiling faces or a spectacular view to remind you of happy moments spent with your camera.

78 Catch it

Ever wondered why you feel so cheerful when you're on vacation, and everyone around you is wearing a big grin? And why are you such a grouch when your nearest and dearest is in a bad mood? The answer is that other people's moods are contagious. Researchers have found that showing people pictures of happy, smiling faces raises levels of brain waves associated with calm and alertness. So, next time you're feeling down, get out your favorite vacation snaps and have a nice browse—just looking at them will make you feel like smiling.

79 Go on, smile!

If you're having a bad day, chances are you are walking around with a face like thunder. Unfortunately, this is how other people will see and react to you, and you can easily get caught up in a complicated chain reaction of bad mood vibes. Yet you can do something astonishingly simple to change all this. All you have to do is smile. It may sound strange, but it's surprisingly effective. The very action of lifting the corners of your mouth into a smile floods the brain with serotonin, a brain chemical that will instantly lift your mood. As a result, you'll give off happier feelings and people will react to you in a more positive way, which will also make you feel good.

80 Let off steam

When you feel really angry your first instinct may be to lash out at the nearest person or object. That's not a good idea. It's much better to let off steam in the great outdoors. Find somewhere quiet and private where you can open your mouth, let rip, and scream to the elements. Yell, stamp your feet, or get a cushion and punch it as hard as you can. Getting rid of stress and pent-up anger this way can be wonderfully energizing, and best of all, it means you don't hurt anyone close to you.

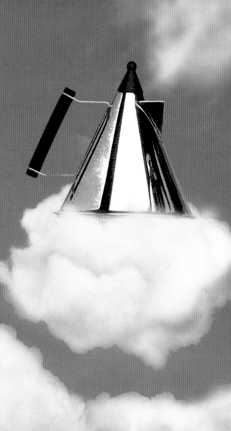

CHAPTER FIVE

happy home

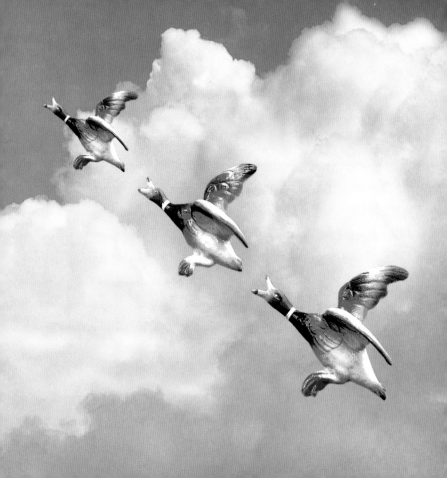

81 Bust that dust

Don't let dust build up in nooks and crannies—it encourages
dust mites and affects the quality of the air in your home. This
can deplete your energy, making it difficult for you to feel positive
and productive. Clean the house regularly to revitalize the
atmosphere. When the sun's shining, take rugs and bedding
outside to air them, clear out cabinets, vacuum carpets at least
once a week, and wash, or dry-clean curtains regularly. Sweep,
wash and polish floors, and wipe down surfaces daily. Invest in a
feather duster for cleaning high corners and pictures.

82 Shaping influences

Think carefully about the atmosphere you want to create in a
room before deciding on how you are going to furnish it. The
shape of the furniture and the material it is made from can affect
the energy balance in your living space. Soft materials such as

wood, bamboo, and wicker in rounded shapes are calming and relaxing. Hard, shiny materials such as ceramic, tile, glass, or marble with angular shapes are more stimulating. The larger the surface area involved, the more intense the effects will be.

83 All fired up

A warmly blazing fire in the fireplace will cheer your heart as well. In addition to being emotionally therapeutic, fires are a great way of circulating air, and the heat they generate is less enervating than central heating. Open fires, with the crackle and smell of burning wood and coals, are intensely evocative. However, simulated log gas fires are also very comforting, and are much easier to clean and maintain. Spaces large and small benefit from the glow of firelight; enjoy an open fire in your bedroom, too. In summer, you can fill the grate with seasonal plants to brighten up the space.

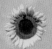

84 Light effects

A dark room with a tiny window can feel most unwelcoming. So how can you transform the area into a really happy space? A few moments of creative thought can solve the problem. All

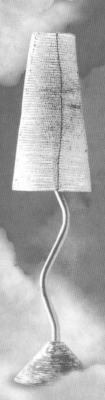

you have to do is paint the walls a
rich, deep color, and fix some recessed spotlights into the ceiling,
ideally on a dimmer switch. Finally, position a few lamps on side
tables, to provide pools of calming light, and you'll have a cozy,
contented retreat where you can escape when things become
too much.

85 Mirror, mirror

Mirrors may be for looking into, but they can also be used to
great effect for reflecting light into a room. It's a classic technique
used by interior decorators. Try placing a really large mirror on a
wall so that it reflects a beautiful view from the outdoors; and
make sure you position it strategically so you can look at the
reflection while sitting in your favorite chair, lying in bed, or even
relaxing in the bath. Remember to keep all your mirrors clean
and bright.

86 Favorite treasures

Surrounding yourself with beautiful objects that you love is a powerful way of creating an uplifting atmosphere in your home. Your chosen treasures may have a special meaning or memory, or you may get pleasure just from looking at them. It's a good idea to group them with a beautiful potted plant or a vase of flowers, to create a natural setting. Every time this display catches your eye, you'll get a rush of positive feeling, which will improve your mood both consciously and unconsciously.

87 Tranquil water

Using water creatively is an ideal way to bring serenity into an inside space. Water trickling from an indoor fountain can mask the sounds of traffic or builder's machinery, and will also refresh the atmosphere of your rooms. Wiping down hard surfaces in the home with water can help to counteract the negative effect of electrical equipment such as televisions or computers. To hydrate a room's atmosphere, place a bowl of water on top of a radiator and introduce extra moisture to your living area with vases of flowers, potted plants, and fish tanks.

88 Sound effects

Sound can either depress or uplift the spirit of your precious living space. Think how a noisy fridge, humming air-conditioner, or a whirring central heating pump can insidiously play on your nerves. Get the problem fixed as soon as possible, before it drains your energy. Sound can be used positively, of course; birdsong and lapping waves are often used for meditation and relaxation and actively lift your spirits. Vigorous sound is also good for enlivening the atmosphere—playing your favorite energetic music while you do the housework will rapidly brighten up the mood of your space.

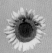

89 Sweet wax

Scented candles work just as well as oil
burners for infusing spaces with pleasing
aromas. Either look out for special ranges, or
create your own with your favorite essential oils.
Burn a chunky pillar candle for a couple of minutes
until it has a pool of melted wax around the
wick. Extinguish the flame, quickly add a couple
of drops of your chosen oil to the wax pool,
then re-light the candle. The wax will be the
correct temperature to release the aroma.
Some oils are flammable, so you should never
add oil to a lighted candle.

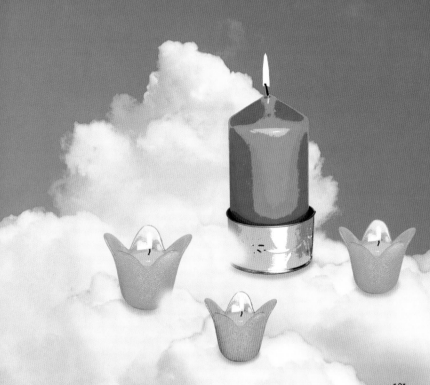

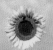

90 Detox the air

Soft furnishings, carpets, paints, and cleaning products can all emit a host of toxic chemicals into the air around you. As a result, you may feel tired and listless. But you can change this. Trials carried out by NASA scientists researching air quality improvements for astronauts showed that common potted plants can detox the air. They absorb poisonous vapors and release oxygen back into the atmosphere. Species to choose include Mexican cacti, spider plants, ivy, rubber plants, and gerbera daisies.

91 Tinkle, tinkle

Hanging wind chimes can enhance the mood of any indoor or outdoor space. In oriental cultures, they have long been used to cleanse and purify the atmosphere. Their intermittent tinkling can have a soft, magical effect, so it is important to choose your wind chime for its sound rather than looks. Play several until you find the notes that please you the most and place it near a window where it will catch the passing breezes.

92 Color and space

When decorating your home, think about the kind of emotional atmosphere you wish to evoke and choose colors accordingly:

- Blue relaxes and calms and is good for rest and communication. It makes a good office color and can help promote a sound night's sleep when used in the bedroom.
- Red uplifts the spirits, but don't overdo it, as the impact can be overpowering.
- Orange is the color of joy and encourages confidence and sociability—it's a good choice for party rooms.
- Yellow is full of vitality and can be used to great effect in kitchens, bathrooms, and work rooms
- Green is the color of balance. Try it in children's rooms.

93 Crystal clear

Placing crystals strategically around your home can help to focus energy. Place them on windowsills where they catch the light, on your desk, or on your computer. Crystals are reputed to have very specific qualities. Try rose quartz for harmony; citrine to build confidence, optimism, and to bring in money; bloodstone for decision-making; carnelian for motivation; clear quartz for focus; amethyst to encourage positive thoughts; jade to help concentration and keep things in perspective; and tiger's eye to enhance your creativity.

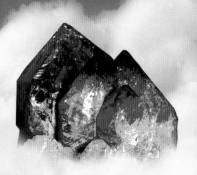

94 Essential influences

Use essential oils imaginatively to change the mood in a room and create the emotional atmosphere you want. Experiment with the following:

- Citrus based oils such as grapefruit, lemon, and orange to refresh, uplift, and invigorate
- Rosemary to clear the air and make you feel more alert
- Peppermint to refresh and stimulate
- Lavender to uplift, calm, and refresh
- Geranium to inspire and invigorate

Add drops of oil to bowls of dried petals or flowers, or use them in an oil burner. Or, try adding a few drops to an atomizer filled with water and spray around the room.

95 Desk top calm

A healthy desk promotes a healthy mind, so introducing order will make you feel more in control, as well as clearer about your priorities. Start by going through your papers, filing them, or throwing them away, as necessary. Keep only work in progress on your desk—this will help to give you mental focus. Look at each paper as it arrives. Either deal with it, file it, or junk it.

96 Ditch the junk

According to ancient Chinese wisdom, clutter represents blocked energy and can quickly bring your spirits down. So, have a good, long think about what is cluttering up your space—whether it's too much furniture, unnecessary equipment, unread newspapers, too many clothes or shoes. Try this formula: if something doesn't lift your mood, or if you haven't used or worn it during the past 12 months, get rid of it or donate it to your local thrift store.

97 Happy paths

Never underestimate the joy-inspiring possibilities of garden paths, flights of steps, patios, or any outside walkways and passages. These areas create a natural breathing space between the interior and the outside world. They should be lovingly nurtured, so you feel on top of the world whenever you are walking through them. Keep these outside areas clean and decorative with pots of colorful, scented flowers and beautiful garden objects.

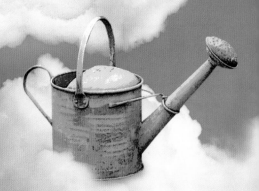

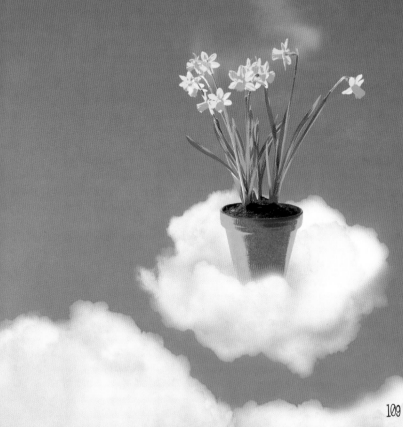

98 Lighten up

Correct lighting can make all the difference to your mood.
Overhead lights can be operated by a dimmer switch, which you
can adjust to suit the moment, and you also need good task
lighting for reading and working. The choice of light bulbs is
important, too. Use full spectrum bulbs (these simulate natural
daylight) in work areas, bathrooms, and kitchens. Natural daylight
bulbs may give a "cold" light, but they are worth considering if
you read a lot. Oil lamps and candles add a soft glow to the
room, but should never be left unattended.

99 Bedroom heaven

It doesn't take much to transform your bedroom into a haven of
peace and tranquillity. Treat yourself to a new bed and pile it up
with pretty cushions. Avoid harsh overhead lights and use the
soft, gentle light of table lamps instead. You could use candles

occasionally, especially those made with pure aromatherapy oils.
It's sheer bliss to fall asleep in a delicately scented room—try
ylang-ylang, sandalwood, or lavender essential oil in a burner, or
put a couple of drops on your pillow. When summer comes, fill a
vase with fresh flowers such as roses, sweet peas, or lilies.

100 Try feng shui

If you're moving home, or renovating your house or apartment,
calling in the feng shui experts could bring a subtle wave of
energy to your new abode. According to this ancient eastern art,
there are hidden energy channels running through the
environment; if these become blocked or stagnant, it can lead to
problems, ranging from lack of money to family arguments. But a
few changes such as clearing out the cabinets, swapping around
the rooms, and careful positioning of furniture can improve the
flow of energy and enhance your health, wealth, and happiness.

acknowledgments

Cover photograph © Images Color Library